LEAN AND HEALTHY

A Comprehensive Guide to Liquid Diets for Weight Loss and Wellness

Adams .U. Morris

TABLE OF CONTENTS

CHAPTER 1

Introduction to Liquid Diets

When we think about food, we often imagine delicious meals on our plates, satisfying our senses and nourishing our bodies. However, there are times when our relationship with food takes a different form, like in the case of liquid diets. This chapter is all about understanding what liquid diets are, why people choose them, the history behind them, and the potential benefits and risks involved.

Defining Liquid Diets

A liquid diet, at its core, is a way of nourishing the body primarily through liquids, as opposed to solid foods. It's a dietary regimen where you consume a variety of fluids that provide essential nutrients, calories, and hydration. These diets can range from simple, clear liquids like water and broth to more complex, nutrient-rich shakes and smoothies.

The Historical Perspective

The concept of liquid diets isn't new; it has been around for centuries in various forms. The idea of consuming liquids for health reasons can be traced back to ancient civilizations. For instance, in ancient Greece, fasting with herbal teas and broths was seen as a way to purify the body and improve overall well-being. Similarly, in Ayurvedic medicine, liquid fasting has been practiced for thousands of years as a means to cleanse the body and promote balance.

Why Liquid Diets?

People turn to liquid diets for a variety of reasons, and it's essential to understand these motivations.

1. **Medical Necessity**: Some individuals may be required to follow liquid diets for medical reasons. This can include preparation for medical procedures, post-surgery recovery, or managing certain medical conditions like gastrointestinal disorders. Clear liquids are often prescribed before surgeries to ensure the digestive tract

is empty and reduce the risk of complications.

2. **Weight Management**: Another common reason is weight loss. Many weight-loss programs incorporate liquid diets as a way to reduce calorie intake and promote rapid weight loss. Liquid diets are often seen as a kickstart to a weight loss journey.

3. **Detoxification**: Liquid detox diets have gained popularity as a means of cleansing the body. These diets typically involve consuming fruit and

vegetable juices for a short period to eliminate toxins and boost overall health.

4. **Convenience**: In today's fast-paced world, liquid diets are also chosen for their convenience. Pre-packaged meal replacement shakes and smoothies offer a quick and easy way to get essential nutrients on the go.

The Potential Benefits

Liquid diets can offer several benefits when used appropriately:

1. **Rapid Weight Loss**: For those looking to shed

pounds quickly, liquid diets can lead to significant initial weight loss due to reduced calorie intake.

2. **Digestive Rest**: Liquid diets can provide the digestive system with a break from the processing of solid foods, which can be helpful for certain medical conditions.

3. **Nutrient Density**: Well-balanced liquid diets can pack a lot of essential nutrients into a small volume, ensuring you get the vitamins and minerals you need.

4. **Hydration**: Liquids help maintain proper hydration, which is crucial for overall health.

The Potential Risks

While liquid diets have their merits, they are not without risks and downsides:

1. **Nutritional Deficiencies**: Extended liquid diets can lead to nutrient deficiencies if not carefully planned. The absence of solid foods can result in a lack of fiber, which is essential for digestive health.

2. **Hunger and Cravings**: It's common to feel hungry and experience cravings on liquid diets, making them challenging to stick to in the long term.

3. **Muscle Loss**: Rapid weight loss from liquid diets can sometimes result in muscle loss along with fat loss.

4. **Metabolic Changes**: Very low-calorie liquid diets can slow down your metabolism, making it harder to maintain weight loss once you return to regular eating.

The Importance of Balance

It's crucial to approach liquid diets with balance and caution. They can be effective tools for specific purposes, but they are not one-size-fits-all solutions. Before embarking on a liquid diet, it's wise to consult with a healthcare professional or registered dietitian. They can help you determine whether a liquid diet is appropriate for your needs and guide you in creating a safe and balanced plan.

In conclusion, liquid diets are a unique approach to nutrition that has been used for centuries for various purposes. They have evolved over time and offer both benefits and risks. The key takeaway from this chapter is that understanding why you are considering a liquid diet and how to use it safely and effectively is essential. It's not just about what you eat or don't eat; it's about nourishing your body in a way that aligns with your specific goals and needs.

This chapter sets the stage for the rest of the book, where we will explore the different types of liquid diets, how to prepare for them, recipes to make them more enjoyable, how to stay nourished, overcome challenges, and consider the health and safety aspects. In the end, our goal is to provide you with the knowledge and tools to make informed decisions about liquid diets and achieve your desired outcomes while prioritizing your health and well-being.

CHAPTER 2

Types of Liquid Diets

In the world of liquid diets, one size certainly does not fit all. There are different types of liquid diets tailored to various needs and circumstances. This chapter aims to shed light on these distinct categories, providing you with a comprehensive understanding of the choices available.

Clear Liquid Diet

Let's start with the simplest and most restrictive form of liquid diet

– the clear liquid diet. This diet is exactly what it sounds like: you consume liquids that are clear, meaning you can see through them. This includes:

1. **Water**: The ultimate clear liquid, keeping you hydrated.

2. **Broth**: Chicken, beef, or vegetable broth provides some flavor and a small amount of nutrients.

3. **Clear Fruit Juices**: Such as apple or white grape juice.

4. **Clear Sports Drinks**: Like Gatorade, to help maintain electrolyte balance.

5. **Clear Tea or Coffee**: Without milk or cream.

6. **Jell-O**: In its clear form, without added fruit or toppings.

A clear liquid diet is often prescribed before medical procedures or surgery. It helps keep the digestive system clear and minimizes residue in the intestines. However, it's extremely low in calories and nutrients, so it's not meant for long-term use.

Full Liquid Diet

A step up from the clear liquid diet is the full liquid diet. This diet includes all the clear liquids plus:

1. **Milk**: Both dairy and non-dairy alternatives like almond or soy milk.

2. **Yogurt**: Plain or flavored, but without solid fruit chunks.

3. **Creamed Soups**: Soups that have been strained to remove solids.

4. **Pudding**: Smooth and creamy pudding is a source of energy.

5. **Custard**: Another calorie-rich option that's easy to swallow.

6. **Ice Cream**: As long as it's fully melted and doesn't contain solid chunks.

The full liquid diet is slightly more nutritionally diverse than the clear liquid diet. It's still often used for short-term periods, especially for individuals who have difficulty chewing or swallowing solid foods, such as those recovering from dental surgery.

Modified Liquid Diet

The modified liquid diet is a more flexible approach. It allows for a combination of clear liquids, full liquids, and additional items such as:

1. **Blended Soups**: Soups that are pureed to a smooth consistency.
2. **Smoothies**: These can be packed with nutrients using ingredients like fruits, vegetables, yogurt, and protein powders.
3. **Mashed Potatoes**: When thinned to a liquid-like consistency.

4. **Oatmeal**: Cooked to a thinner texture.

This type of liquid diet is often used as a transitional phase between full liquids and a regular solid diet. It's more balanced in terms of nutrition and can be adapted to meet individual dietary requirements.

Detox and Juice Cleanses

Detox diets, also known as juice cleanses, have gained popularity in recent years. These diets typically involve consuming freshly squeezed fruit and vegetable juices for a specified period, usually a few days to a week. The idea is to "cleanse" the body of toxins and promote overall health.

Juice cleanses can provide an abundance of vitamins, minerals, and antioxidants from the fruits and vegetables used. However, there are some important considerations:

1. **Lack of Fiber**: Juices lack the fiber found in whole fruits and vegetables, which is essential for digestive health.

2. **Calorie Intake**: While juices are nutritious, they can be low in calories, which

may not be suitable for long-term use or for those with high energy needs.

3. **Sustainability**: Some argue that the detoxification claims of juice cleanses are not scientifically supported.

4. **Potential for Overconsumption**: It's easy to consume a lot of sugar (albeit natural) when drinking fruit juices, which can affect blood sugar levels.

Juice cleanses can be a refreshing way to increase your intake of fruits and vegetables, but they are best used intermittently rather than as a long-term diet.

Medically Supervised Liquid Diets

Lastly, there are medically supervised liquid diets. These are highly specialized diets designed and monitored by healthcare professionals. They are often used for specific medical conditions or extreme weight loss situations. Two common examples include:

1. **Very Low-Calorie Diets (VLCDs)**: These diets provide a limited number of calories, typically under 800

per day. They are usually reserved for individuals with severe obesity under close medical supervision.

2. **Ketogenic Liquid Diets**: These diets are designed to induce a state of ketosis, where the body burns fat for energy. They are used for certain medical conditions, such as epilepsy or as part of a weight loss program.

Medically supervised liquid diets should only be undertaken with the guidance of a healthcare provider due to their potential risks and need for ongoing monitoring.

In summary, there's a wide spectrum of liquid diets to choose from, ranging from clear liquids to medically supervised plans. The type of liquid diet you should consider depends on your specific goals and circumstances. Before embarking on any liquid diet, it's crucial to consult with a healthcare professional or registered dietitian to ensure that it aligns with your nutritional needs and is safe for you. Remember, the key is not just the type of diet but how it's used and for what purpose, as each

serves a unique role in the realm
of nutrition.

CHAPTER 3

Preparing for a Liquid Diet

Embarking on a liquid diet requires more than just swapping out solid foods for liquids. It involves careful planning, mental preparation, and gathering the necessary resources. This chapter guides you through the steps to take before you start your liquid diet, ensuring you're set up for success.

1. Consultation with a Healthcare Professional

Before making any significant dietary changes, it's vital to consult with a healthcare professional. This could be your primary care doctor, a registered dietitian, or a nutritionist. They can evaluate your health status, assess your dietary needs, and help you determine whether a liquid diet is appropriate for you. If you have underlying health conditions, are pregnant, or are taking certain medications, their guidance is especially important.

2. Define Your Goals

Clearly defining your goals for the liquid diet will guide your approach. Are you looking to lose weight, prepare for a medical procedure, or simply detox your body? Understanding your motivations will help you select the most suitable type of liquid diet and set realistic expectations.

3. Creating a Personalized Liquid Diet Plan

Once you've discussed your goals with a healthcare professional, work together to create a personalized liquid diet plan. This plan should align with your nutritional needs, preferences, and any dietary restrictions you might have. It's essential that the plan provides adequate calories, essential nutrients, and hydration to support your body's functions.

4. Setting Realistic Goals

Set achievable goals that are specific, measurable, and time-bound. For instance, if weight loss is your aim, determine how much weight you intend to lose and over what period. Keep in mind that very rapid weight loss through extreme calorie restriction may not be sustainable in the long run and could have negative health consequences.

5. Gathering Supplies and Ingredients

Preparing for a liquid diet means having the right supplies and ingredients on hand. This might include:

- **Blender or Juicer**: Depending on the type of liquid diet you're following, a blender or juicer could be essential for creating smoothies or fresh juices.

- **Storage Containers**: You'll need containers to store prepared liquids, such as soups, broths, or shakes.

- **Reusable Straws**: These can be helpful for sipping liquids without having to use a spoon.

- **Nutrient-Rich Ingredients**: Stock up on fruits, vegetables, protein powders, and other ingredients that will provide a well-rounded nutrient profile.

6. Psychological Preparation

Transitioning to a liquid diet can be mentally challenging, especially if you're used to eating solid foods. Take some time to mentally prepare yourself for the journey:

- **Mindset Shift**: Understand that the purpose of a liquid diet is to nourish your body, and it's a temporary phase.

- **Support System**: Inform your friends and family about your decision to follow a liquid diet. Having their support can be immensely helpful, especially when you encounter challenges.

- **Mindful Eating**: Be prepared to practice mindful eating even with liquids. Savor the flavors and textures of the liquids you consume.

7. Meal Planning and Prep

As with any diet, planning and preparation are key. Plan your meals ahead of time, considering your daily schedule and activities. This will help you stay on track and avoid last-minute temptations.

8. Gradual Transition

If you're switching from a regular diet to a liquid one, consider gradually reducing solid foods. This can help your body adjust more smoothly to the change.

9. Educate Yourself

Take time to educate yourself about the nutritional aspects of your chosen liquid diet. Understanding the types of nutrients you'll be consuming will help you make informed decisions and prevent deficiencies.

10. Seek Emotional Support

Changing your diet can sometimes trigger emotional responses. If you find yourself struggling emotionally, consider seeking support from a therapist or counselor. They can help you navigate any challenges or feelings that may arise during this transition.

In conclusion, preparing for a liquid diet is about more than just choosing the right foods. It involves understanding your body's needs, setting realistic goals, gathering necessary supplies, and mentally preparing for the journey ahead. Taking the time to plan and consult with healthcare professionals ensures that your liquid diet experience is safe, effective, and aligned with your overall well-being.

This chapter sets the foundation for the rest of your liquid diet journey. As you move forward, remember that patience, flexibility, and self-care are essential companions on this path. With the right preparation, you'll be better equipped to face challenges and embrace the benefits of a well-planned liquid diet.

CHAPTER 4

Liquid Diet Recipes

A liquid diet doesn't have to be bland or monotonous. In this chapter, we'll explore a variety of liquid diet recipes that not only meet your nutritional needs but also tantalize your taste buds. From nutrient-rich smoothies to hearty soups, these recipes will help you navigate your liquid diet with flavor and variety.

1. Nutrient-Rich Smoothie Recipes

Smoothies are a staple of many liquid diets because they can be packed with essential nutrients. Here are some recipes to get you started:

- **Green Power Smoothie**:
    - Ingredients: Spinach, kale, banana, Greek yogurt, almond milk, and honey.
    - Instructions: Blend all ingredients until smooth. This provides a dose of leafy greens and protein.
- **Berry Blast Smoothie**:

- o Ingredients: Mixed berries (strawberries, blueberries, raspberries), yogurt, almond milk, and a touch of honey.
  - o Instructions: Blend until creamy for a fruity and antioxidant-rich treat.
- **Tropical Delight Smoothie**:
  - o Ingredients: Pineapple, mango, coconut milk, and a scoop of protein powder.

- o Instructions: Blend for a taste of the tropics and a protein boost.

2. Homemade Soups and Broths

Soups and broths can provide warmth and comfort on your liquid diet journey. Here are a couple of recipes to try:

- **Classic Chicken Broth**:
  - o Ingredients: Chicken broth, a pinch of salt, and a dash of black pepper.
  - o Instructions: Warm the broth, season to

taste, and sip slowly. This is gentle on the stomach and soothing.

- **Creamy Tomato Soup**:
  - Ingredients: Tomato juice, a touch of olive oil, basil, salt, and pepper.
  - Instructions: Combine the ingredients, heat, and garnish with fresh basil for a tomato soup alternative.

3. Vegetable and Fruit Juices

Freshly squeezed juices are a fantastic way to get a burst of vitamins and minerals. Here are a couple of juice recipes:

- **Carrot-Apple-Ginger Juice**:
  - Ingredients: Carrots, apples, a small piece of ginger.
  - Instructions: Run the ingredients through a juicer for a zesty, vitamin-rich juice.
- **Mean Green Juice**:
  - Ingredients: Kale, cucumber, green apple, lemon, and a touch of mint.

o   Instructions: Juice the ingredients for a refreshing and nutrient-packed green juice.

4.   Protein-Packed   Liquid Meals

If you're concerned about protein intake, these recipes offer a boost:

- **Protein Shake**:
    - o   Ingredients: Protein powder (whey, pea, or plant-based), almond milk, a banana, and a tablespoon of almond butter.

- o Instructions: Blend for a protein-rich, creamy shake.

- **Quinoa and Vegetable Puree**:

  - o Ingredients: Cooked quinoa, steamed vegetables (e.g., broccoli, carrots), vegetable broth.

  - o Instructions: Blend the ingredients until smooth for a protein and fiber-rich meal.

5. Tips for Flavor and Variety

To add flavor and variety to your liquid diet, consider these tips:

- **Herbs and Spices**: Experiment with herbs like basil, cilantro, and mint, and spices such as ginger, cinnamon, and cayenne pepper to enhance the taste of your liquids.

- **Citrus Zest**: Grate a bit of lemon, lime, or orange zest into your liquids for a burst of fresh citrus flavor.

- **Fruit Infusions**: Add slices of fruits like cucumber, lemon, or berries to your water for natural flavor.

- **Protein Options**: Explore different protein sources such as whey, soy, pea, or collagen protein powders to find what suits your taste.

- **Texture**: Vary the texture of your liquids by blending them for different lengths of time. A shorter blend time will result in a chunkier texture, while longer blending will create a smoother consistency.

6. Portion Control

On a liquid diet, it's crucial to pay attention to portion control. Even though you're consuming liquids, you can still overdo it on calories and nutrients. Use measuring cups or a kitchen scale to ensure you're meeting your dietary goals without excess.

7. Timing Matters

Consider the timing of your liquid meals. Spread them evenly throughout the day to keep your energy levels stable and prevent hunger pangs. Some people find it helpful to have small, frequent meals, while others prefer fewer, larger meals.

8. Stay Hydrated

Don't forget to drink water in addition to your liquid meals. Staying hydrated is essential for overall health. You can infuse your water with slices of lemon, cucumber, or mint for added flavor.

9. Adjust to Your Preferences

These recipes are starting points. Feel free to modify them to suit your preferences and nutritional needs. You can adjust sweetness levels, spice levels, or even switch out ingredients to keep things fresh and exciting.

10. Get Creative

Liquid diets can be a culinary adventure. Don't hesitate to get creative with your recipes. Try new combinations of fruits, vegetables, and other ingredients to discover flavors you enjoy.

In conclusion, a liquid diet doesn't mean sacrificing taste and variety. With the right recipes and a bit of creativity, you can enjoy a diverse range of flavors and nutrients while adhering to your liquid diet plan. Remember that the key to success on a liquid diet is not only the nutritional content of your meals but also the pleasure you derive from them. By exploring these recipes and adapting them to your taste, you can make your liquid diet a satisfying and enjoyable experience.

CHAPTER 5

Staying Nourished on a Liquid Diet

Switching to a liquid diet doesn't mean compromising on nutrition. In fact, it's crucial to ensure that you're getting all the essential nutrients your body requires to function optimally. This chapter provides insights into meeting your nutritional needs, monitoring calorie intake, staying hydrated, considering supplements and vitamins, and avoiding common deficiencies while on a liquid diet.

Meeting Nutritional Requirements

One of the primary concerns on a liquid diet is making sure you receive all the necessary nutrients. Here's how to approach it:

- **Balanced Liquid Meals**: Ensure that each liquid meal contains a mix of macronutrients—carbohydrates, proteins, and fats—as well as essential vitamins and minerals. This balance is key to overall health.
- **Variety Is Key**: Incorporate a wide range of

ingredients into your liquid recipes. Different fruits, vegetables, and protein sources will help you cover various nutrients.

- **Fiber Matters**: Although liquid diets often lack fiber, try to incorporate some sources of soluble fiber like psyllium husk or flaxseed to support digestive health.

- **Monitor Your Intake**: Keep track of your daily nutrient intake to ensure you're meeting your dietary goals. You might find apps or nutrition calculators useful for this.

Monitoring Calorie Intake

Calorie intake is a crucial aspect of any diet, including liquid diets. It's essential to balance your caloric intake with your energy expenditure, whether you're aiming for weight loss or maintenance. Here's how to manage calorie intake on a liquid diet:

- **Calorie Counting**: Be mindful of your calorie consumption. Liquid diets can vary significantly in calorie content, so tracking your intake will help you achieve your goals.

- **Don't Go Too Low**: While calorie reduction is often a goal in weight loss, extremely low-calorie diets can slow down your metabolism and lead to muscle loss. It's important to strike a balance.

- **Consult a Dietitian**: If you're unsure about your calorie needs or how to calculate them, consider consulting a registered dietitian. They can provide personalized guidance based on your goals and health status.

Hydration and Fluid Balance

Maintaining proper hydration is vital for overall health, and this doesn't change on a liquid diet. In fact, because you're consuming more liquids, you may need to pay extra attention to hydration:

- **Water Intake**: In addition to the liquids that make up your meals, continue to drink plain water throughout the day to stay adequately hydrated.

- **Electrolyte Balance**: Some liquid diets, especially those that involve significant fluid loss, may affect your electrolyte balance. Consult with a healthcare provider to ensure that your electrolytes remain in check.

- **Monitor Urine Color**: A simple way to gauge your hydration status is to observe the color of your urine. Light yellow or pale straw is generally a sign of good hydration, while dark yellow may indicate dehydration.

Supplements and Vitamins

Liquid diets can sometimes fall short in providing all the vitamins and minerals your body needs.

Here's how to address potential deficiencies:

- **Consult with a Healthcare Provider**: Talk to your healthcare provider or a registered dietitian about the potential need for supplements. They can recommend appropriate options based on your diet and health status.

- **Multivitamins**: In some cases, a daily multivitamin or mineral supplement can help bridge nutritional gaps. However, supplements should not be used as a replacement for whole foods.

- **Regular Monitoring**: While on a liquid diet, have regular check-ups with your healthcare provider to monitor your nutritional status. Blood tests can help identify deficiencies early.

Avoiding Common Deficiencies

On a liquid diet, you may be at risk of certain deficiencies due to the absence of solid foods. Here are some common deficiencies to watch out for:

- **Protein**: Ensure that your liquid diet includes adequate protein sources to prevent muscle loss. Protein is essential for maintaining and repairing body tissues.

- **Vitamin B12**: If you're not including animal products in your liquid diet, you may be at risk of vitamin B12 deficiency. Consider fortified foods or supplements if needed.

- **Calcium**: Liquid diets may lack calcium, which is vital for bone health. Look for calcium-fortified liquids or talk to your healthcare provider about supplements.

- **Folate**: Ensure your diet includes folate-rich ingredients, especially if you're pregnant or planning to become pregnant.

- **Iron**: If your liquid diet doesn't include sources of heme iron (found in animal products), you might need to pay attention to iron intake. Iron supplements may be necessary, but consult a healthcare provider before taking them.

- **Vitamin D**: Depending on your sun exposure and

dietary choices, you might need to consider vitamin D supplements, as it is challenging to obtain sufficient vitamin D from a liquid diet alone.

Conclusion

In summary, staying nourished on a liquid diet requires careful planning and attention to your nutritional needs. Whether you're following a liquid diet for medical reasons or weight management, it's essential to prioritize your health. This chapter highlights the importance of balanced liquid meals, monitoring calorie intake, staying hydrated, considering supplements and vitamins, and avoiding common deficiencies.

A liquid diet can be a valuable tool when used correctly and with proper guidance from healthcare professionals. Remember that the key to success on a liquid diet is not only achieving your dietary goals but also maintaining your overall well-being. By making informed choices, monitoring your health, and seeking professional guidance, you can ensure that your liquid diet journey is both effective and safe.

CHAPTER 6

Overcoming Challenges

Transitioning to a liquid diet, whether for medical reasons or weight management, can be a rewarding but challenging journey. In this chapter, we'll explore some of the common obstacles people face while on a liquid diet and offer practical strategies to help you overcome them.

1. Dealing with Hunger and Cravings

Challenge: One of the most significant challenges of a liquid diet is dealing with hunger and food cravings, especially in the initial stages when your body is adjusting to the new eating pattern.

Solution:

- **Frequent, Small Meals**: Instead of sticking to a traditional three-meals-a-day schedule, consider having smaller, more frequent liquid meals. This can help keep hunger at bay.
- **Stay Hydrated**: Sometimes, thirst is

mistaken for hunger. Drink water or herbal tea between your liquid meals to stay hydrated and curb unnecessary snacking.

- **High-Fiber Liquids**: Include liquids with some fiber content, such as blended vegetable soups or smoothies with added ground flaxseeds. Fiber can help you feel fuller for longer.
- **Mindful Eating**: Pay close attention to the flavors, textures, and aromas of your liquid meals. This can help satisfy your senses and

reduce the desire for solid foods.

2. Managing Social Situations

Challenge: Social gatherings and events often revolve around food, making it challenging to stick to your liquid diet plan and participate fully in such occasions.

Solution:

- **Communicate**: Inform your friends and family about your dietary restrictions. Most people are understanding and willing to accommodate your needs.

- **Plan Ahead**: If possible, offer to bring your own liquid meal or drink to social events. This way, you can enjoy the company without feeling pressured to eat solid foods.

- **Focus on Socializing**: Shift the focus of social gatherings away from food. Engage in conversations, games, or activities to distract yourself from the temptation to eat.

3. Coping with Emotional Aspects

Challenge: Food is often intertwined with emotions, and not being able to eat solid foods can lead to emotional challenges like frustration, sadness, or even guilt.

Solution:

- **Seek Support**: Talk to a therapist or counselor if you're struggling emotionally. They can help you address any emotional issues related to your diet.
- **Practice Mindfulness**: Engage in mindfulness techniques to manage emotional eating. When you

feel an urge to eat for emotional reasons, take a moment to breathe and reflect on your feelings.

- **Journaling**: Keeping a journal can be therapeutic. Write down your thoughts and emotions related to your liquid diet journey to gain clarity and perspective.

4. Adhering to the Diet Plan

Challenge: Staying committed to a liquid diet, especially over an extended period, can be challenging due to monotony or the desire for solid foods.

Solution:

- **Variety**: Experiment with different liquid recipes to keep your meals interesting and satisfying. Variety can prevent diet fatigue.

- **Set Realistic Goals**: Ensure that your diet plan is sustainable in the long term. If you find it too restrictive, work with a healthcare professional to adjust it to your needs.

- **Support System**: Lean on your support system, whether it's friends, family, or online communities.

Sharing your challenges and achievements can help you stay motivated.

5. Avoiding Potential Pitfalls

Challenge: Liquid diets can have pitfalls, such as not meeting nutritional requirements or compromising your health if not followed correctly.

Solution:

- **Consult a Professional**: Before starting a liquid diet, consult with a healthcare provider or registered dietitian. They can help you create a safe and balanced plan.

- **Regular Check-ups**: If you're on a long-term liquid diet, schedule regular check-ups with your healthcare provider to monitor your health and nutritional status.

- **Transition Gradually**: If you plan to transition back to solid foods, do so gradually under the guidance of a healthcare professional. This can help prevent digestive issues.

6. Achieving Long-Term Success

Challenge: Maintaining the benefits of a liquid diet over the long term can be challenging, especially if you revert to unhealthy eating habits afterward.

Solution:

- **Transition Plan**: Work with a registered dietitian to create a transition plan. This should outline how you'll reintroduce solid foods while maintaining a balanced diet.

- **Lifestyle Changes**: Use the knowledge gained during your liquid diet journey to make lasting lifestyle changes. Focus on incorporating healthy eating habits into your daily life.

- **Monitor Your Progress**: Continue to monitor your weight, energy levels, and overall well-being after your liquid diet. Regular self-assessment can help you stay on track.

Conclusion

While a liquid diet can present various challenges, it's important to remember that with the right strategies and support, you can successfully navigate these obstacles. Dealing with hunger, managing social situations, coping with emotional aspects, adhering to the diet plan, avoiding pitfalls, and achieving long-term success all require careful planning, perseverance, and sometimes, seeking professional guidance.

Your liquid diet journey is not just about short-term goals; it's an opportunity to develop a healthier relationship with food, improve your dietary habits, and prioritize your well-being. By addressing these challenges head-on and staying committed to your goals, you can make your liquid diet experience not only successful but also personally transformative.

Remember, you have the capacity to overcome challenges and achieve your desired outcomes while prioritizing your health and happiness.

CHAPTER 7

Health and Safety Considerations

Safety should always be a top priority when undertaking any dietary regimen, including liquid diets. In this chapter, we'll delve into key health and safety considerations to ensure that your liquid diet journey is both effective and safe.

1. Consultation with Healthcare Professionals

Consideration: Before embarking on a liquid diet, it's imperative to consult with healthcare professionals. This includes your primary care physician and, ideally, a registered dietitian.

Importance: Healthcare professionals can assess your overall health, any underlying medical conditions, and determine whether a liquid diet is appropriate for you. They can also help create a personalized plan tailored to your needs and monitor your progress along the way.

2. Duration and Purpose of the Diet

Consideration: Define the purpose and duration of your liquid diet. Is it for weight loss, medical reasons, or detoxification? Is it a short-term cleanse or a long-term dietary change?

Importance: Clarifying the purpose and duration of your liquid diet will guide your approach and help set realistic expectations. For example, very low-calorie liquid diets designed for rapid weight loss may not be suitable for long-term use.

3. Proper Hydration

Consideration: Staying hydrated is essential. Ensure that your liquid diet provides adequate fluids, and continue to drink plain water throughout the day.

Importance: Proper hydration is crucial for overall health and well-being. It supports bodily functions, including digestion, circulation, and temperature regulation. Dehydration can lead to a range of health issues and should be avoided.

4. Nutritional Adequacy

Consideration: A well-balanced liquid diet should provide essential nutrients, including carbohydrates, proteins, fats, vitamins, and minerals.

Importance: Nutritional adequacy is essential to avoid deficiencies and promote overall health. Lack of nutrients can lead to fatigue, muscle loss, and other health complications. Work with a registered dietitian to ensure your liquid diet meets your nutritional needs.

5. Monitoring and Adjustment

Consideration: Regular monitoring of your progress and health status is vital. Pay attention to factors like weight, energy levels, and any symptoms or discomfort.

Importance: Monitoring allows you to make necessary adjustments to your diet plan. If you experience adverse effects or nutrient deficiencies, healthcare professionals can intervene promptly to address these issues.

6. Avoid Extreme Calorie Restriction

Consideration: Very low-calorie liquid diets, especially those below 800 calories per day, can be extreme and should be used cautiously.

Importance: Extremely low-calorie diets can slow down your metabolism, lead to muscle loss, and have adverse health effects. It's crucial to strike a balance between calorie reduction for weight loss and maintaining your body's essential functions.

7. Physical Activity

Consideration: Determine your physical activity level and how it fits into your liquid diet plan.

Importance: Exercise is an essential component of a healthy lifestyle. Consult with healthcare professionals to ensure that your physical activity aligns with your liquid diet goals and doesn't compromise your health.

8. Recognize Signs of Malnutrition

Consideration: Be aware of the signs and symptoms of malnutrition, which can include

fatigue, weakness, hair loss, and
brittle nails.

Importance: Malnutrition can
occur if your liquid diet lacks
essential nutrients. Recognizing
the signs early allows for timely
intervention and adjustments to
your dietary plan.

9. Gradual Transition

Consideration: If you plan to
transition from a liquid diet back
to solid foods, do so gradually.

Importance: Gradual transition
helps your digestive system adapt
to solid foods again, reducing the

risk of digestive discomfort and other issues.

10. Psychological Well-being

Consideration: Pay attention to your mental and emotional well-being throughout your liquid diet journey.

Importance: The psychological aspect of dieting is significant. If you experience emotional distress, seek support from a therapist or counselor to help you manage any challenges that arise.

11. Listen to Your Body

Consideration: Tune in to your body's signals and adjust your diet accordingly.

Importance: Your body knows best when it comes to hunger and fullness cues. Pay attention to how you feel and make dietary choices accordingly.

12. Individualization

Consideration: Recognize that not all liquid diets are suitable for everyone. Your dietary plan should be personalized to your unique needs and circumstances.

Importance: What works for one person may not work for another.

Individualization ensures that your diet aligns with your health goals, preferences, and any medical conditions you may have.

13. Potential Risks and Contraindications

Consideration: Be aware of potential risks and contraindications associated with certain liquid diets.

Importance: Some individuals, such as pregnant or breastfeeding women, those with certain medical conditions, or individuals with a history of eating disorders, may not be suitable candidates for specific types of liquid diets. Consulting with healthcare professionals helps identify these risks.

14. Reintroducing Solid Foods

Consideration: If your liquid diet is temporary, plan how you will reintroduce solid foods when the diet period ends.

Importance: A well-planned transition can help prevent digestive discomfort and allow you to resume a balanced diet more comfortably.

15. Long-Term Goals

Consideration: Consider your long-term health and dietary goals beyond the liquid diet.

Importance: A liquid diet is often a temporary phase. Think about how you will maintain the health benefits achieved during the diet and what dietary habits you'll adopt moving forward.

Conclusion

In conclusion, health and safety considerations are paramount when undertaking a liquid diet. The guidance of healthcare professionals, careful planning, proper hydration, nutritional adequacy, monitoring, and addressing potential challenges all play a vital role in ensuring that your liquid diet journey is both effective and safe.

Remember that a liquid diet should prioritize your health and well-being above all else. With proper guidance and attention to these considerations, you can embark on your liquid diet journey confidently, knowing that you are taking steps to safeguard your health while working toward your dietary and health goals.

CHAPTER 8

Transitioning Out of a Liquid Diet

Transitioning out of a liquid diet is a crucial phase that requires careful planning and consideration. After following a liquid diet for a specific purpose, such as weight loss or a medical procedure, it's essential to reintroduce solid foods gradually and mindfully. This chapter outlines the steps and strategies for a successful transition.

1. The Importance of Gradual Transition

Consideration: Gradual transition is key to a successful return to solid foods after a liquid diet.

Importance: Your digestive system needs time to readjust to processing solid foods. A sudden shift can lead to discomfort, digestive issues, and even shock to your body. Gradual transition minimizes these risks.

2. Consult with a Healthcare Professional

Consideration: Always consult with your healthcare provider or a registered dietitian before starting the transition phase.

Importance: They can provide personalized guidance based on your health status, dietary preferences, and the type of liquid diet you followed. They may also conduct assessments to ensure you're ready for solid foods.

3. Determine the Right Timing

Consideration: Timing is crucial when transitioning out of a liquid diet.

Importance: The length of your liquid diet, your specific health goals, and any medical procedures you've undergone all influence the timing. Your healthcare provider can help determine the best time to start transitioning.

4. Selecting the First Solid Foods

Consideration: Begin with easily digestible and low-fiber foods.

Importance: Foods like plain cooked rice, steamed vegetables, or lean proteins are gentle on your digestive system. They're less likely to cause discomfort or digestive issues during the initial transition phase.

5. Portion Control

Consideration: Be mindful of portion sizes, especially in the early days of transitioning.

Importance: Your stomach has likely shrunken during the liquid diet, so overeating can lead to discomfort. Start with small portions and listen to your body's hunger and fullness cues.

6. Maintain Hydration

Consideration: Continue to prioritize hydration as you reintroduce solid foods.

Importance: Staying well-hydrated supports digestion and overall health. Don't forget to drink water between meals.

7. Pay Attention to Your Body

Consideration: Be attuned to how your body responds to different foods.

Importance: Some foods may be better tolerated than others. Pay attention to any signs of discomfort or adverse reactions and adjust your diet accordingly.

8. Gradually Increase Fiber Intake

Consideration: Slowly introduce higher-fiber foods as your digestive system adapts.

Importance: Fiber is essential for digestive health, but a sudden increase can cause bloating and discomfort. Incorporate foods like whole grains, beans, and fruits gradually.

9. Monitor Digestive Health

Consideration: Keep an eye on your digestive health during the transition.

Importance: If you experience persistent digestive issues or discomfort, consult with your healthcare provider. They can offer guidance and assess if any underlying issues need addressing.

10. Avoid Highly Processed Foods

Consideration: Stay away from heavily processed or high-sugar foods during the transition.

Importance: Processed foods can be harsh on your digestive system and may not provide the nutrients your body needs for recovery.

11. Balanced Diet Reintegration

Consideration: Gradually reintegrate a variety of food groups into your diet.

Importance: A balanced diet provides essential nutrients. Aim to include a mix of carbohydrates, proteins, healthy fats, and a wide range of fruits and vegetables.

12. Individualization

Consideration: Your transition plan should be tailored to your unique needs and preferences.

Importance: What works for one person may not work for another. Your healthcare provider or dietitian can help you create a plan that aligns with your goals and health status.

13. Listen to Your Body

Consideration: Tune in to your body's signals throughout the transition.

Importance: Your body will provide feedback on what foods work well and what causes discomfort. Pay attention and adjust your diet accordingly.

14. Dietary Modifications

Consideration: If you have specific dietary restrictions or preferences, incorporate them into your transition plan.

Importance: A transition plan that aligns with your dietary needs is more likely to be sustainable in the long term.

15. Mindful Eating

Consideration: Practice mindful eating during the transition.

Importance: Eating mindfully helps you savor your food, recognize hunger and fullness cues, and make conscious food choices.

16. Continue Monitoring

Consideration: Maintain regular check-ins with your healthcare provider or dietitian even after the transition phase.

Importance: Ongoing monitoring ensures that you're progressing as planned and that your dietary choices align with your long-term health goals.

17. Reestablishing Healthy Eating Habits

Consideration: Use the transition phase as an opportunity to reestablish healthy eating habits.

Importance: Your liquid diet journey may have provided insights into your relationship with food. Incorporate these lessons into your regular eating habits for long-term well-being.

18. Celebrate Achievements

Consideration: Celebrate your achievements and progress.

Importance: Recognize the milestones you've reached and the positive changes you've made to your diet and health. Celebrating achievements can be motivating and reinforce healthy habits.

19. Seek Support

Consideration: Lean on your support system when needed.

Importance: The transition phase can come with its challenges. If you encounter difficulties or have questions, don't hesitate to seek support from friends, family, or healthcare professionals.

CONCLUSION

Transitioning out of a liquid diet is a crucial phase that should be approached with careful planning and consideration. Gradual reintroduction of solid foods, consultation with healthcare professionals, timing, portion control, hydration, and mindful eating are all vital aspects of a successful transition. By following these considerations and listening to your body, you can navigate this phase smoothly and ensure a healthy return to regular eating habits while maintaining the benefits of your liquid diet journey.